COMPLETE GUIDE TO GASTROINTESTINAL PERFORATION

A Comprehensive Medical Resource For Understanding Causes, Symptoms, Diagnosis, And Treatment

DEHART HAIRSTON

© [DEHART HAIRSTON], [2024]

All rights reserved. No part of this publication may be reproduced, distributed, or transmitted in any form or by any means, including photocopying, recording, or other electronic or mechanical methods, without the prior written permission of the publisher, except in the case of brief quotations embodied in critical reviews and certain other noncommercial uses permitted by copyright law.

DISCLAIMER

This book's content is only intended for general informative purposes. At the time of writing, the author has taken every precaution to guarantee that the material is correct and current. Nevertheless, the author disclaims all explicit and implicit representations and guarantees about the availability, appropriateness, correctness, completeness, and usefulness of the material on these pages.

Since the author is not a licensed medical practitioner, the material in this book shouldn't be interpreted as medical advice. Before making any modifications to their diet, exercise regimen, or medical treatment, readers are urged to speak with a licensed healthcare provider.

Moreover, the author has no connection to any of the businesses, organizations, or people that are discussed in this book. Any mentions of goods, services, businesses, or people are purely informative and do not indicate endorsement or suggestion.

This book's content is entirely dependent on the author's expertise, study, and comprehension of the topic. Despite having taken reasonable care to offer correct information, the author disclaims all liability for any mistakes or omissions in the material as well as for any losses, harm, or damages resulting from using the information.

It is recommended that readers use their own judgment and discretion when applying the knowledge in this book to their own situations. The use or implementation of any material in this book may result in unfavorable repercussions, directly or indirectly, for which the author assumes no liability.

By reading this book, you agree to release and hold the author harmless from any claims, losses, liabilities, costs, or expenditures resulting from or related to the use of the information you get from it.

Table of Contents

CHAPTER 1 13
- Understanding Gastrointestinal Perforation 13
- What Is Gastrointestinal Perforation? 13
- Causes And Risk Factors 14
- Symptoms and Indications 16

CHAPTER 2 19
- Anatomy Of The Digestive System 19
- Overview Of The Digestive Tract 19
- Key Structures Involved 20
- Function Of Each Digestive Organ 21

CHAPTER 3 25
- Types Of Gastrointestinal Perforation 25
- Differentiating Between Types 25
- Location-Based Perforations 27
- Severity And Complications 29

CHAPTER 4 33
- Diagnosis Of Gastrointestinal Perforation 33
- Clinical Evaluation 33
- Diagnostic Tests And Imaging 35
- Importance Of Early Detection 37

CHAPTER 5 41
Treatment Options 41
Immediate Care In Emergency Settings 41
Surgical Interventions 43
Non-Surgical Approaches 45

CHAPTER 6 47
Post-Treatment Care And Recovery 47
Hospital Stay And Follow-Up Visits 47
Rehabilitation And Dietary Guidelines 49
Monitoring For Complications 51

CHAPTER 7 53
Prevention Strategies 53
Lifestyle Modifications 53
Recognizing Warning Signs 55
High-Risk Groups And Precautions 56

CHAPTER 8 59
Complications And Long-Term Effects 59
Potential Complications After Treatment 59
Management Of Long-Term Effects 61
Quality Of Life Considerations 62

CHAPTER 9 65

Patient Perspectives And Support 65
Coping Strategies 65
Peer Support Networks 66
Resources For Patients And Families 68
CHAPTER 10 71
Future Directions And Research 71
Advancements In Treatment Methods 71
Emerging Technologies 74
Areas Of Ongoing Research 76
CONCLUSION 80
THE END 83

ABOUT THE BOOK

For anybody worried about digestive health, "Gastrointestinal Perforation: A Comprehensive Guide" is an invaluable resource. This well-written book explores the complex realm of gastrointestinal perforation, including information on causes, symptoms, diagnosis, available treatments, and long-term effects. Let's examine the reasons why your medical library has to include this book.

"Gastrointestinal Perforation" provides a comprehensive grasp of the ailment itself, first and foremost. By explaining the idea of gastrointestinal perforation, its many causes, and related risk factors, Chapter 1 establishes the foundation. The next chapters include professional details on the signs and symptoms, which you must recognize with this core knowledge. Understanding these foundational concepts is essential for early identification and intervention, regardless of whether you work in healthcare or are just a concerned citizen.

In addition, Chapter 2 of the book offers a thorough synopsis of the digestive system's anatomy. Comprehending the complexity of gastrointestinal perforation requires an understanding of the fundamental structures and the complicated workings of the digestive system. This section provides readers with the necessary information to navigate the subtleties of the illness by explaining the role of each digestive organ.

The focus on diagnosis and therapy in this book is one of its most notable aspects. The several gastrointestinal perforation diagnostic procedures, imaging modalities, and treatment choices are covered in detail in Chapters 4 and 5. The book provides vital insights on properly treating this severe condition, ranging from urgent treatment in emergency settings to surgical and non-surgical approaches.

Furthermore, "Gastrointestinal Perforation" addresses post-treatment care, rehabilitation, and preventative techniques in addition to therapy approaches. To reduce the chance of a recurrence, Chapters 6 and 7 include recommendations on hospital stays, follow-up visits, rehabilitation, food instructions, and lifestyle changes.

Crucially, the book delves into the human side of the issue in addition to the clinical components. Chapter 9 explores peer support networks, coping mechanisms, patient viewpoints, and patient and family resources. For comprehensive patient management, it is crucial to understand the psychological effects of gastrointestinal perforations.

Finally, Chapter 10's "Gastrointestinal Perforation" provides an outlook on the next studies and developments. To keep readers up to date on the most recent advancements in the industry, the book highlights areas of active study as well as upcoming technology.

Gastrointestinal Perforation: A Comprehensive Guide" is an invaluable resource for patients, caregivers, and medical professionals. Its all-encompassing information, practical insights, and holistic approach make it an invaluable resource for anybody navigating the challenges of gastrointestinal health. This book is a priceless tool that you just cannot afford to ignore, whether your goal is to improve patient care or broaden your knowledge.

CHAPTER 1

Understanding Gastrointestinal Perforation

What Is Gastrointestinal Perforation?

A disorder known as a "gastrointestinal perforation" is characterized by a hole or tear in the gastrointestinal tract's wall. The esophagus, stomach, small intestine, and large intestine (colon) are all parts of this system. If this hole is not addressed right once, it may cause the contents and digestive fluids to flow into the abdominal cavity, which might result in serious consequences.

Several factors, including underlying medical issues or physical trauma, may cause the perforation. It's critical to recognize that gastrointestinal perforation is a medical emergency that has to be treated right away to stop further problems.

Causes And Risk Factors

Gastrointestinal perforation may be caused by several reasons, including:

1. Peptic Ulcers: These are open sores that appear on the top portion of the small intestine or the inside lining of the stomach. Peptic ulcers have the potential to perforate the digestive system if they are not treated, wearing down the wall.

2. Diverticulitis: Diverticula are tiny, protruding pouches that may develop in the digestive tract's lining, usually the colon. Diverticulitis is a disease caused by inflammation or infection of these pouches. The diverticula may burst in extreme circumstances, resulting in perforation.

3. Gastric cancer: Tumorous growths in the stomach have the potential to erode the stomach wall's strength and raise the possibility of a perforation.

4. IBD stands for inflammatory bowel disease. Disorders such as Crohn's disease and ulcerative colitis may irritate and damage the lining of the digestive system, increasing the risk of a perforation.

5. Physical Trauma: The gastrointestinal system may puncture itself directly as a result of blunt force trauma or penetrating abdominal injuries.

6. Iatrogenic Causes: If some medical procedures, including colonoscopies or endoscopies, are not done appropriately, they may unintentionally result in perforation.

Advanced age, a history of gastrointestinal issues, smoking, heavy alcohol use, and long-term use of corticosteroids or nonsteroidal anti-inflammatory medicines (NSAIDs) are risk factors for gastrointestinal perforation.

Symptoms and Indications

Depending on the location and extent of the hole, different gastrointestinal perforations might present with different signs and symptoms. On the other hand, typical symptoms might be:

- **Sudden and Severe Abdominal Pain:** Depending on where the perforation occurs, this pain is often quite severe and may be either localized or widespread.

- **Nausea and Vomiting:** Patients may have ongoing nausea and vomiting, and their vomit may include blood as well.

- **Abdominal Tenderness and stiffness:** Peritonitis, or inflammation of the abdominal lining, is characterized by tenderness to the touch and stiffness or guarding of the abdominal muscles.

- **Fever and chills:** An infection brought on by a perforation may cause these symptoms.

- **Reduced Bowel Sounds:** When the abdomen is auscultated, medical professionals may notice diminished or nonexistent bowel sounds.

If you encounter any of these symptoms, you must get medical help right away since a gastrointestinal perforation left untreated may result in potentially fatal outcomes including organ failure, sepsis, and the development of an abscess. For a good result, early diagnosis and action are essential.

CHAPTER 2

Anatomy Of The Digestive System

Overview Of The Digestive Tract

The gastrointestinal (GI) tract, often referred to as the digestive tract, is a sophisticated mechanism that breaks down and absorbs nutrients from the food we eat. Saliva and chewing start the process of digestion in the mouth, and it continues to the anus, where waste products are eliminated from the body.

Several specialized organs and structures are involved in the passage of food through the digestive system, and each is vital to the process. The mouth, esophagus, stomach, small intestine, large intestine (colon), rectum, and anus are among these organs. Every organ has a different role in the digestive process as a whole.

Key Structures Involved

1. Mouth: The digestive system enters the body via the mouth. Here, chewing breaks down food mechanically and combines it with saliva, which includes enzymes that start the chemical digestion process.

2. Esophagus: The muscular tube that joins the mouth and stomach is known as the esophagus. Its main job is to move food from the mouth to the stomach by contracting the muscles in a motion known as peristalsis.

3. Stomach: The digesting process that begins in the mouth is carried out in the stomach, a very acidic organ. It secretes gastric juices, which further break down food into chyme, a semi-liquid material. These secretions include hydrochloric acid and enzymes.

4. Small Intestine: The bulk of nutrition absorption occurs in the small intestine. It is divided into the ileum, jejunum, and duodenum. Vitamins, proteins, lipids, and carbs are all broken down and absorbed with the help of pancreatic enzymes and liver bile.

5. Large Intestine (Colon): The colon is the part of the body that forms feces by collecting water and electrolytes from the residual indigestible food. Additionally, a sizable colony of beneficial bacteria resides there, helping to promote the fermentation of undigested carbohydrates.

6. Rectum and Anus: During defecation, the rectum acts as a holding area for waste products until they are ejected from the body via the anus.

Function Of Each Digestive Organ

- **Mouth:** Food is broken down into smaller bits by chewing, which increases the surface area available for enzyme activity. Enzymes like amylase, which are found in saliva, start the breakdown of carbohydrates.

- **Esophagus:** Using a rhythmic contraction process known as peristalsis, the esophagus moves food efficiently and reflux-free from the mouth to the stomach.

- **Stomach:** The stomach produces digestive fluids that include pepsin, an enzyme that breaks down proteins into smaller peptides, and hydrochloric acid. It also acts as a food reservoir, controlling how much food enters the small intestine.

- **Small Intestine:** The main location of nutrition absorption is the small intestine. Proteins, carbs, and lipids are more easily absorbed when bile from the liver and pancreas is combined with enzymes from the pancreas to enhance the surface area for absorption.

- **Large Intestine (Colon):** The gut bacteria create vitamins, electrolytes, and water that the colon absorbs. Additionally, before feces are released from the body, it retains and compacts them.

- **Rectum and Anus:** Until defecation, waste products are stored in the rectum. The anal sphincters regulate the body's excretion process, making sure it occurs at the right time and location.

CHAPTER 3

Types Of Gastrointestinal Perforation

Differentiating Between Types

A hazardous medical ailment known as a "gastrointestinal perforation" occurs when a hole opens up in the wall of the stomach, small intestine, or large intestine. To properly diagnose and treat gastrointestinal perforations, one must be aware of their many kinds. These kinds may be distinguished by several variables, such as the severity of the ailment, the location of the perforation, and the source.

The location of the hole may be used to distinguish between various forms of gastrointestinal perforations. For example, a hole in the stomach is called a gastric perforation, but an intestinal perforation is the name given to a hole in the small intestine. In a similar vein, a large intestine hole is referred to as a colonic perforation. various treatment modalities may be needed for each kind of perforation, since they may exhibit various symptoms.

The etiology of the hole should be taken into account while distinguishing between various forms of gastrointestinal perforations. Numerous conditions, including trauma, ulcers, infections, and certain medical treatments, may result in perforations. While perforations brought on by ulcers may be the consequence of chronic inflammation or infection, traumatic perforations may be the consequence of blunt force trauma or piercing injuries to the abdomen. If left untreated, infections like diverticulitis or appendicitis may potentially result in gastrointestinal perforation.

Furthermore, the kind of gastrointestinal perforation might affect how severe the illness is. Certain holes are tiny and isolated, resulting in few symptoms and necessitating conservative care; other perforations are bigger and more widespread, posing a serious risk of serious consequences including sepsis or peritonitis. The possibility of complications and the urgency of treatment will depend on how severe the perforation is.

Location-Based Perforations

Gastrointestinal perforations that happen in certain parts of the digestive system are referred to as location-based perforations. The stomach, small intestine, or large intestine may all sustain these perforations, and each poses unique difficulties and treatment options.

Peptic ulcers, gastric cancer, and abdominal trauma are among the illnesses that are often linked to gastric perforations, which are holes in the stomach. A stomach perforation may cause excruciating pain in the abdomen, nausea, vomiting, and shock symptoms including low blood pressure and a fast heartbeat. Imaging tests like X-rays or CT scans are often used to diagnose stomach perforations. Surgical closure of the hole and the administration of antibiotics to avoid infection are possible treatments.

The small intestine may become perforated due to several illnesses such as diverticulitis, Crohn's disease, or abdominal trauma. Fever, bloating, constipation, and stomach discomfort are some signs of intestinal perforation. An endoscopy or CT scan may be used to diagnose intestinal perforations, and surgery to close the wound and remove any injured tissue may be the course of therapy.

Large intestine perforations, or colonic perforations, are often linked to diseases such as diverticulitis, colorectal cancer, or inflammatory bowel disease. A colonic perforation may cause fever, sepsis-like symptoms, rectal bleeding, and abdominal discomfort. Imaging tests like CT scans or colonoscopies may be used to diagnose colonic perforations, and surgery to close the hole and remove any damaged colon tissue may be the course of therapy.

Severity And Complications

The size, location, etiology, and general health of the patient are some of the variables that might affect the severity of a gastrointestinal perforation. Perforations may vary in size and cause life-threatening consequences. In some instances, they are tiny and asymptomatic.

Peritonitis, which happens when bacteria from the digestive system enter the abdominal cavity via the hole and cause inflammation and infection of the peritoneum, the membrane lining the abdominal cavity, is one of the primary problems linked to gastrointestinal perforations. Severe stomach pain, fever, nausea, vomiting, and shock symptoms including low blood pressure and a fast heartbeat are all possible outcomes of peritonitis. To treat peritonitis, surgery is usually required to close the perforation and remove any contaminated tissue. Antibiotics are also often used to manage the infection.

Sepsis, which happens when the body's immunological response to an infection becomes dysregulated and causes extensive inflammation and organ failure, is another consequence of gastrointestinal perforation. Sepsis has to be treated right away since it might be fatal.

Sepsis treatment may include antibiotics to treat the underlying infection along with supportive care such as IV fluids, oxygen therapy, and drugs to sustain blood pressure and organ function.

In addition to bowel obstruction, fistula development, abscess formation, and systemic problems such as organ failure and mortality, gastrointestinal perforations may also result in several other issues. The underlying cause of the perforation, the patient's general health, and the promptness of detection and treatment all affect the likelihood of complications. For patients with gastrointestinal perforations, lowering the risk of sequelae and enhancing outcomes are contingent upon early detection and care.

CHAPTER 4

Diagnosis Of Gastrointestinal Perforation

Clinical Evaluation

The first step in detecting gastrointestinal perforation, a dangerous medical disease that needs immediate care, is clinical assessment. To ascertain the probability of a gastrointestinal perforation, medical experts closely evaluate the patient's symptoms, medical history, and physical examination results during the clinical assessment.

Individuals who have had gastrointestinal perforation often exhibit acute abdomen, a condition marked by intense and sometimes abrupt abdominal pain. Usually confined, this discomfort may become worse as you move or palpate it. Abdominal distension, fever, nausea, and vomiting are other typical symptoms.

Medical professionals must get a thorough history of the patient's symptoms, including when they first appeared, how severe they were, and any triggers or mitigating variables.

Healthcare professionals evaluate the patient's symptoms as well as conduct a comprehensive physical examination. To detect regions of tenderness, stiffness, or guarding—all of which may point to peritoneal irritation and perhaps signal the possibility of a gastrointestinal perforation—they may palpate the abdomen. Additional symptoms including tympany, rebound soreness, or a palpable lump may also be helpful in the diagnosis process.

All things considered, the clinical assessment is critical in helping to diagnose gastrointestinal perforation since it offers valuable details about the patient's physical findings and symptoms. Healthcare professionals may establish the need for further diagnostic testing and imaging investigations to confirm the diagnosis and direct the proper course of treatment by carefully examining these results.

Diagnostic Tests And Imaging

To diagnose gastrointestinal perforation, diagnostic tests, and imaging investigations are crucial tools that aid medical professionals in determining the site of the hole, verifying its existence, and monitoring it for potential consequences such as abscess development or peritonitis. Depending on the perforation's presumed etiology and clinical presentation, a variety of diagnostics and imaging modalities may be used.

Abdominal X-rays are among the most often used diagnostic procedures for gastrointestinal perforations. The primary indicator of a hole, free air in the peritoneal cavity, may be promptly found with this imaging technique.

Free air gives a visible sign of perforation on an X-ray by appearing as radiolucent regions beneath the diaphragm or around the intestinal loops. Because abdominal X-rays are easily accessible and provide quick findings, they are often the first imaging examination carried out in patients who have a suspected gastrointestinal perforation.

Patients with suspected gastrointestinal perforation may also be evaluated using ultrasonography and computed tomography (CT) scans in addition to an abdominal X-ray. The specific position and extent of the perforation, as well as the detection of sequelae like abscesses or fistulas, may all be determined using a CT scan. In specific situations, ultrasound may be employed, such as in individuals who may have gynecological or appendicitis-related perforations.

In general, imaging examinations and diagnostic tests are crucial for the diagnosis of gastrointestinal perforation because they tell medical professionals about the existence, location, and severity of the hole and help them make choices regarding subsequent treatment. Healthcare professionals may guarantee that patients with this potentially fatal illness get prompt and appropriate therapy by carefully evaluating the findings of these tests.

Importance Of Early Detection

Improving patient outcomes and lowering the risk of consequences require early diagnosis of gastrointestinal perforations. A digestive tract perforation is a medical emergency that has to be treated right away to avoid serious side effects including sepsis, multi-organ failure, and peritonitis. As a result, medical professionals need to be on the lookout for gastrointestinal perforation symptoms and indications and act quickly to start the proper diagnosis and treatment.

The possibility of quick clinical deterioration in individuals with gastrointestinal perforations is one of the main arguments in favor of early identification. If medical attention is delayed, a perforation may allow stomach contents or feces to seep into the peritoneal cavity, resulting in infection and severe inflammation. This may lead to peritonitis, a dangerous sickness marked by fever, chills, and symptoms similar to a systemic illness. Severe instances of peritonitis may proceed quickly, resulting in organ failure, septic shock, and even death.

Early identification of gastrointestinal perforation not only prevents problems from developing but also enables the beginning of suitable treatment. Treatment options include surgical repair, antimicrobial treatments, and supportive measures including fluid resuscitation and pain management, depending on the underlying cause and degree of the perforation. Healthcare professionals may improve patient outcomes and lower the likelihood of long-term consequences by promptly delivering therapies for gastrointestinal perforation when it is diagnosed.

All things considered, it is crucial to identify gastrointestinal perforations as soon as possible. Healthcare practitioners may prevent complications from this critical medical disease and maximize patient outcomes by identifying the signs and symptoms of perforation early on and starting the necessary diagnostic and therapeutic steps right away.

CHAPTER 5

Treatment Options

Immediate Care In Emergency Settings

In the event of a gastrointestinal perforation, immediate medical intervention is critical. Stabilizing the patient and taking care of any potentially fatal consequences are the main priorities in emergencies. As soon as the patient arrives, the medical staff will do a comprehensive evaluation to determine the amount of the perforation and how it may affect the patient's health. This evaluation may involve a physical examination, imaging tests like X-rays or CT scans, and laboratory testing.

Resuscitation techniques are often used in immediate care to restart essential bodily processes including breathing and circulation. Intravenous fluids and blood transfusions may be given to a patient exhibiting indications of shock as a result of internal bleeding or infection to sustain blood pressure and oxygen supply to critical organs.

In situations when it is believed that the perforation resulted from an external item or trauma, such as a gunshot wound or blunt force trauma, immediate surgery can be required to fix the damage and stop future consequences. Another essential component of prompt treatment is pain control, which reduces suffering and enhances the patient's general health.

Close observation of the patient's vital signs and symptoms is necessary throughout the emergency treatment procedure to identify any changes or problems as soon as possible. To maximize the patient's chances of a favorable result, emergency doctors, surgeons, nurses, and other healthcare professionals work together to guarantee a coordinated and efficient response to gastrointestinal perforation situations.

Surgical Interventions

To adequately heal gastrointestinal perforations, surgery is often necessary. The precise surgical technique is determined by several variables, including the size and location of the hole, the underlying etiology, and the patient's general health.

An exploratory laparotomy, in which the abdomen is surgically opened to directly see and heal the hole, is a popular surgical technique for gastrointestinal perforations. The surgeon closely inspects the abdominal organs throughout the process to look for any new wounds or issues and treats them as necessary.

Primary closure, in which the perforation's margins are sutured together to close the hole, may be used when the perforation is little and isolated. More involved surgical procedures, such as resection and anastomosis, in which the damaged piece of the intestine is removed and the remaining healthy ends are rejoined, may be necessary for bigger or polluted holes.

A temporary diverting stoma may be made in some cases, especially if the perforation is the result of a severe infection or inflammation, to give the afflicted section of the intestine time to recover. To redirect the flow of feces away from the location of the hole, part of the intestine must be brought to the surface of the belly.

For gastrointestinal perforations, post-operative care is essential to achieving the best possible recovery and avoiding complications. This might include treating pain, using antibiotics to stop infections, and providing dietary assistance to speed up the healing process. Throughout the postoperative phase, the patient's status is closely monitored to spot any early warning indicators of problems including bleeding, infection, or intestinal blockage.

Non-Surgical Approaches

When it comes to minor holes or individuals who are not good candidates for surgery because of underlying medical issues, non-surgical methods of managing gastrointestinal perforations may be taken into consideration in some situations.

Conservative therapy is a non-surgical technique in which the patient is kept under careful observation in a hospital environment and is given supportive care, including intravenous fluids, antibiotics, and pain relief. To avoid the necessity for surgery and let the perforation heal itself is the aim of conservative therapy.

Endoscopic treatment is another non-surgical strategy that could be used in certain situations. To reach the perforation site, a flexible tube called an endoscope—which is connected to a camera and surgical instruments—is introduced via the mouth or rectum. To stop bleeding or seal minor wounds, endoscopic methods including suturing, cutting, or adding sealants might be used instead of open surgery.

It's crucial to remember, nevertheless, that not all people with gastrointestinal perforations may benefit from non-surgical methods. A case-by-case analysis should be conducted to determine if non-surgical care is warranted, including variables such as the extent and position of the perforation, the underlying etiology, and the patient's general state of health.

Throughout non-surgical therapy, careful observation of the patient's state is crucial, with frequent evaluations to gauge the success of the selected course of action and to quickly identify any indications of problems.

CHAPTER 6

Post-Treatment Care And Recovery

Hospital Stay And Follow-Up Visits

Your hospital stays and follow-up appointments after gastrointestinal perforation therapy are essential parts of your healing process. You'll get medical attention and careful monitoring during your hospital stay to guarantee the best possible healing and recuperation.

You will probably go through several diagnostic tests when you are admitted to the hospital to evaluate the severity of the perforation and choose the best course of action. Depending on how serious your situation is, you could need surgery to close the perforation, or you might only need to take supportive care and antibiotics.

You will be under constant observation by medical staff members, including physicians, nurses, and other specialists, while you are in the hospital. Your vital signs will be routinely evaluated, any infections or other problems will be watched for, and your treatment plan will be modified as necessary.

Apart from medical attention, you may need help with everyday living tasks and pain treatment to ensure your comfort throughout your hospital stay, especially if you have had surgery. It's critical that you adhere to your doctor's recommendations and let them know right away if anything changes with your health.

Following your hospital release, your doctor will probably have follow-up appointments set up for you to check on your recuperation and make sure everything is going according to plan. To evaluate healing and identify any possible issues, these follow-up appointments may include laboratory testing, imaging scans, and physical exams.

It is imperative that you show up for these follow-up appointments if you want your treatment to be successful and to avoid difficulties on the road. Together, you and your healthcare provider will create a customized follow-up care plan that is suited to your unique requirements and situation.

Rehabilitation And Dietary Guidelines

After a gastrointestinal perforation, rehabilitation is essential to your recovery, especially if you've had surgery or seen a substantial reduction in your physical ability. To help you restore your strength, mobility, and independence, rehabilitation programs may involve physical therapy, occupational therapy, and nutritional counseling.

Through focused exercises and activities, physical therapy aims to increase your physical strength, flexibility, and endurance. Your physical therapist may create a personalized rehabilitation program to address any functional limits or mobility challenges you may be having based on your requirements.

The goal of occupational therapy is to assist you in regaining the knowledge and skills required to carry out everyday tasks like cooking, cleaning, and clothing. For you to do these chores more independently, your occupational therapist could give assistive technology or teach you adaptive skills.

Optimizing your nutritional intake and promoting recovery after a gastrointestinal perforation needs dietary coaching. You may need to adhere to a certain diet or avoid certain foods to prevent problems like intestinal blockage or discomfort, depending on the location and severity of the perforation.

A certified dietician or your healthcare physician may provide recommendations on dietary changes that are specific to your requirements and interests. They could suggest consuming more of certain nutrients to aid in healing and steering clear of items that might aggravate pain or symptoms related to the digestive system.

Monitoring For Complications

Following gastrointestinal perforation therapy, it's critical to keep an eye out for any issues that can develop during the healing phase. Infection, the development of an abscess, intestinal blockage, and recurrence of the hole are a few examples of complications.

Your doctor will give you advice on what symptoms to look out for and when to get in touch with them if you have any alarming ones. Fever, elevated abdominal discomfort or soreness, nausea or vomiting, altered bowel habits, and trouble passing gas or stool are a few examples.

During the healing process, it's critical to take care of your emotional and mental health in addition to keeping an eye out for any medical difficulties. It may be difficult to manage a significant medical condition such as gastrointestinal perforation, and you may feel a variety of feelings such as worry, anxiety, and frustration.

Gaining assistance from loved ones, friends, or mental health specialists may be beneficial in managing these psychological obstacles and advancing general healing and wellness. Recovering is a prolonged process, so keep that in mind, and don't be afraid to take each day as it comes, concentrating on little victories and benchmarks along the road.

CHAPTER 7

Prevention Strategies

Lifestyle Modifications

A major factor in avoiding stomach perforation is changing one's lifestyle. Keeping up a healthy diet is one important component. Consuming a well-balanced diet full of fruits, vegetables, lean meats, and fiber will help to maintain digestive health and lower the chance of ailments like constipation, which can exacerbate perforation. Limiting alcohol and caffeine intake, as well as avoiding overindulging in spicy or acidic meals, may all improve digestive health.

A crucial lifestyle change is drinking enough water. By consuming enough water, one may avoid problems like dehydration and constipation and maintain the digestive system's optimal operation. Although it's advised to consume eight glasses of water or more each day, each person's requirements may differ depending on their age, amount of exercise, and climate.

Exercise regularly is also crucial for preserving digestive health. By promoting digestion and bowel motions, physical exercise lowers the risk of constipation and other digestive issues. To promote overall digestive function, try to get in at least 30 minutes of moderate activity most days of the week.

Furthermore, maintaining gastrointestinal health might benefit from stress management. Prolonged stress may harm digestion and raise the possibility of disorders like peptic ulcers, which, if addressed, might rupture. Deep breathing exercises, yoga, meditation, and other stress-reduction methods may enhance gut health and encourage calm.

Recognizing Warning Signs

To avoid gastrointestinal perforation, early warning sign detection might be very important. For timely medical intervention, it is important to recognize the signs of disorders such as peptic ulcers, diverticulitis, or inflammatory bowel disease that might result in perforation.

Abdominal discomfort or cramping, bloating, changes in bowel habits (constipation or diarrhea), nausea, vomiting, and rectal bleeding are common indicators of gastrointestinal problems. It is imperative that you get medical assistance as soon as possible if you develop any of these symptoms, particularly if they are severe or persistent.

More severe symptoms, such as abrupt and intense stomach pain, fever, chills, fast pulse, trouble breathing, and indicators of shock (pale complexion, fast breathing, and dizziness), may sometimes be brought on by gastrointestinal perforations. These signs may point to a medical emergency and call for prompt medical intervention.

Frequent visits to the doctor may also aid in detecting and treating any gastrointestinal problems that may be present before they become severe enough to cause a perforation. Individual risk factors and medical history may dictate the recommendation for routine screens and diagnostic testing, such as colonoscopies or endoscopies.

High-Risk Groups And Precautions

There may be a larger risk of gastrointestinal perforation in some groups of people, thus additional care should be taken to avoid this dangerous consequence. Individuals who have already had gastrointestinal disorders such as diverticulitis, Crohn's disease, or inflammatory bowel disease are more vulnerable and should adhere to their doctor's advice while treating these problems.

Regular users of nonsteroidal anti-inflammatory medicines (NSAIDs), such as aspirin or ibuprofen, should exercise additional caution since these drugs increase the risk of perforations and ulcers in the gastrointestinal tract. To reduce this risk, use NSAIDs as prescribed and refrain from high-dose or prolonged usage.

Due to age-related changes in the digestive system, the existence of other medical disorders, and the use of drugs, older persons constitute another high-risk population for gastrointestinal perforation. Senior citizens must be in constant contact with their healthcare practitioner and report any new or worrisome symptoms as soon as possible.

Because these conditions may raise the risk of complications, those who have had previous abdominal operations or injuries to the abdomen should also be especially watchful for symptoms of gastrointestinal perforation. It is possible to promote appropriate healing and lower the risk of problems by adhering to post-operative care instructions and making follow-up consultations with a surgeon or other healthcare professional.

To avoid gastrointestinal perforation and promote digestive health, it is important to be aware of personal risk factors, maintain a healthy lifestyle, recognize warning signals, and seek medical assistance promptly when necessary.

CHAPTER 8

Complications And Long-Term Effects

Potential Complications After Treatment

A dangerous ailment, intestinal perforation needs immediate medical care and suitable treatment to avoid complications. Even with the greatest of intentions on the part of medical professionals, problems may sometimes occur during or after treatment. Infection is one possible side effect. A perforation in the gastrointestinal system may allow intestinal germs to seep into the abdominal cavity, where they can cause peritonitis, an infection of the cavity's lining. Severe stomach pain, fever, nausea, and vomiting are some of the symptoms that may be caused by peritonitis. To manage the infection and stop additional problems, prompt treatment with antibiotics and potentially surgery may be required.

Sepsis, a potentially fatal illness that arises when the body's reaction to an infection results in extensive inflammation, is another possible consequence of gastrointestinal perforation. If left untreated, sepsis may result in organ failure and even death. Sepsis is more likely to occur in patients with gastrointestinal perforations, especially if the rupture is not identified and treated right once. For these individuals to have better results, sepsis must be identified early and aggressively managed.

Abscesses, or pockets of pus that occur as a result of infection, may sometimes result from gastrointestinal perforations. Symptoms of an abscess might include fever, chills, and discomfort in the abdomen. To treat an abscess, it is usually necessary to drain it surgically or with the use of image-guided methods like CT or ultrasound scanning. It is also possible to administer antibiotics to help treat the illness.

Management Of Long-Term Effects

Patients may have long-term complications from gastrointestinal perforations that need to be managed even if therapy is effective. Adhesions, or the formation of scar tissue in the abdomen, are a typical long-term consequence. In some situations, adhesions may result in symptoms including infertility, intestinal blockage, and persistent abdominal discomfort. Dietary changes, painkillers, and, in some situations, surgery to remove scar tissue are all possible treatments for adhesions.

Malnutrition is another possible long-term consequence of gastrointestinal perforation. Malnutrition might eventually result from damage to the gastrointestinal system, which can hinder the body's capacity to absorb nutrients from meals.

To make sure they are getting enough nutrients, patients may need to change their diet or take nutritional supplements.

Gastrointestinal perforations may significantly affect a patient's emotional and psychological health in addition to their physical problems. Having a chronic illness and managing its symptoms may be difficult, and it can make you feel depressed, anxious, or alone in society. To assist patients deal with the long-term repercussions of gastrointestinal perforation, healthcare professionals should address these psychological elements of treatment and provide tools and support.

Quality Of Life Considerations

For those who have had gastrointestinal perforations, maintaining a high quality of life is crucial. This entails attending to social and emotional needs in addition to physical issues.

Together, patients and healthcare professionals should create a thorough care plan that takes into consideration each patient's unique preferences and objectives.

A key component of helping individuals with gastrointestinal perforations live better lives is pain management. Persistent stomach discomfort may significantly affect everyday activities and general health. Pain management and quality-of-life enhancement strategies may include a mix of pharmaceuticals, physical therapy, and other treatments administered by healthcare professionals.

To treat the psychological and emotional effects of gastrointestinal perforation, supportive care is also essential. To assist patients deal with the difficulties of having a chronic illness, counseling, support groups, or other psychological therapies may be beneficial. Patients' quality of life may also be enhanced by encouraging them to continue with social activities and hobbies.

In general, a thorough and multidisciplinary strategy is needed to manage the long-term consequences and difficulties of gastrointestinal perforation. Healthcare professionals may assist patients to maximize their quality of life and achieve better results by attending to both the physical and emotional components of treatment.

CHAPTER 9

Patient Perspectives And Support

Coping Strategies

Patients often experience feelings of helplessness and uncertainty when confronted with the severe problem of gastrointestinal perforation. Coping mechanisms are essential for assisting people in getting through this trying period with fortitude and resiliency. Asking for help from family members and medical experts is a useful coping technique. Patients might find consolation and security in knowing that they are not alone on their path by candidly sharing their worries and anxieties.

A helpful coping technique is to have an optimistic mindset and concentrate on the things in life that make you happy and fulfilled. Anxiety and hopelessness may be lessened by partaking in relaxing and stress-reduction activities like yoga, meditation, and outdoor recreation. Furthermore, patients who are well-informed about their ailment and available treatments are better equipped to actively engage in their healthcare choices, which promotes their feeling of agency and control.

Moreover, embracing wholesome lifestyle practices like consistent exercise, a balanced diet, and enough sleep may enhance general well-being and fortitude in the face of difficulty. When used regularly and intentionally, these coping mechanisms may offer patients the fortitude and stamina required to overcome the difficulties associated with gastrointestinal perforation.

Peer Support Networks

Peer support networks are a great resource for those dealing with gastrointestinal perforations as they provide support, empathy, and encouragement. Making connections with others who have gone through comparable circumstances may provide coping mechanisms, helpful advice, and a feeling of validation and belonging. Through social media networks, online forums, or in-person support groups, patients may find comfort in sharing their experiences and ideas with others who get what they're going through.

Peer support networks facilitate the exchange of information on gastrointestinal perforation management, including treatment choices, healthcare providers, and resources. Through the pooling of other patients' experiences and collective knowledge, people might get important viewpoints and insights that would not be easily obtained via conventional medical channels.

Peer support networks can provide patients with a feeling of advocacy and empowerment, enabling them to actively participate in their treatment process. People may influence positive change in the healthcare system and increase access to high-quality treatment for gastrointestinal perforations in themselves and others by speaking out for their needs and concerns.

Resources For Patients And Families

When negotiating the complications of gastrointestinal perforation, patients and their families need to have access to extensive information. A vast array of resources are available to aid people in making educated choices and overcoming obstacles, ranging from educational materials and internet resources to financial assistance programs and support services.

Educational resources on the causes, symptoms, diagnosis, and treatment of gastrointestinal perforation include booklets, brochures, and web articles. With the help of these materials, patients and their families will be better able to comprehend their situation and interact with medical professionals.

Financial aid programs have the potential to mitigate the financial strain incurred by medical charges, including hospital bills, prescription drugs, and continuous treatment fees. Patients may avoid the additional stress of financial difficulty by investigating available options and asking for help when required. This allows patients to concentrate on their rehabilitation.

Furthermore, patients and their families may get emotional and psychological assistance from support services including peer support groups, counseling, and therapy as they manage the highs and lows associated with gastrointestinal perforations. These services provide a supportive and secure space where people may express their emotions, look for advice, and find comfort in the company of others who have been through similar experiences.

Through the efficient use of these tools, patients and their families may get the necessary support and guidance to successfully manage the problems associated with gastrointestinal perforation and begin the process of healing and recovery.

CHAPTER 10

Future Directions And Research

Advancements In Treatment Methods

Improvements in therapy techniques have completely changed patient outcomes and care in the field of gastrointestinal perforations. Historically, the main method of treating perforations has been surgery, which involves open procedures and long recovery periods. However, patients now have access to less invasive procedures with faster recovery times because of the development of minimally invasive methods like robotic surgery and laparoscopy.

Laparoscopic surgery, sometimes referred to as "keyhole surgery," involves creating tiny abdominal incisions through which specialized tools and a camera are placed.

Compared to conventional open surgery, this enables doctors to precisely see and fix holes, resulting in less discomfort after surgery, shorter hospital stays, and quicker recovery. Similar to this, robotic-assisted surgery makes use of sophisticated robotic devices that are managed by surgeons to carry out difficult operations with more accuracy and dexterity.

The creation of tissue adhesives and sealants represents a noteworthy improvement in therapeutic techniques. In some situations, these materials may be applied directly to the perforation site to seal the defect and encourage tissue repair, doing away with the requirement for staples or sutures. Tissue adhesives have the benefit of reducing tissue damage and speeding up the healing process, especially when surgery is difficult or dangerous.

The treatment of gastrointestinal perforation has greatly benefited from developments in medicinal therapy as well as advances in surgery. Proton pump inhibitors assist in lower stomach acid output, which promotes faster healing of perforations, whereas antibiotics are often used to prevent and treat infections related to perforations. Additionally, improvements in nutritional assistance and intensive care management have helped patients with gastrointestinal perforations heal more fully and live better overall.

Further innovation and refinement in treatment options for gastrointestinal perforations is possible as long as medical science and technology keep developing. To maximize the therapy of this difficult illness, physicians and researchers are always looking for novel methods and strategies to improve patient outcomes, lower complications, and raise overall survival rates.

Emerging Technologies

The diagnosis and treatment of gastrointestinal perforations are changing due to emerging technology, which provides new opportunities for better patient outcomes. Endoscopic suturing is one such method that allows medical professionals to seal holes using an endoscope without the need for invasive surgery. In addition to lowering the dangers involved with open surgery, this minimally invasive method enables speedier recovery periods and shorter hospital stays.

The development of sophisticated imaging modalities, such as contrast-enhanced computed tomography (CT) scans and magnetic resonance imaging (MRI), is another hopeful technological advancement. With the use of these imaging methods, perforations and the surrounding tissues may be seen in great detail, improving diagnosis and treatment planning.

These technologies help physicians identify and locate perforations early on, which allows them to act quickly and efficiently to reduce the risk of complications and enhance patient outcomes.

Moreover, the discipline of regenerative medicine has the potential to completely transform the way gastrointestinal perforations are treated. Improved healing of holes may result from tissue engineering approaches that encourage tissue regeneration and repair, such as the use of scaffolds seeded with stem cells. These novel treatments may improve patients' long-term results from gastrointestinal perforations by using the body's natural ability to regenerate.

Emerging technologies are changing the landscape of research and development in the area of gastrointestinal perforation in addition to technical developments in treatment approaches. In a virtual setting, researchers may investigate intricate physiological processes and refine therapeutic approaches thanks to sophisticated computer models and simulation tools. Researchers may find new biomarkers and therapeutic targets by using big data analytics and machine learning algorithms. This opens the door for customized medicine methods that are catered to the specific requirements of each patient.

These cutting-edge technologies have the potential to completely transform the identification, management, and course of therapy for gastrointestinal perforations, providing both patients and medical professionals with fresh hope as they develop and mature.

Areas Of Ongoing Research

Even though gastrointestinal perforation diagnosis and therapy have gone a long way, there are still a lot of research projects underway that try to improve patient outcomes and deepen our knowledge of this complicated illness. The creation of new biomarkers for the early diagnosis and risk assessment of perforations is one area of concentration. To create non-invasive diagnostic tools that can precisely forecast and track the course of the illness, researchers are working to uncover distinct biomolecular fingerprints linked to the development of perforations.

The investigation of alternative therapeutic techniques, such as targeted medication delivery systems and regenerative treatments, is another area of active study. Stem cell-based strategies have the potential to minimize long-term consequences and lessen the need for surgical intervention by encouraging tissue regeneration and repair in ruptured organs. In a similar vein, the creation of tailored drug delivery systems enables the localized distribution of therapeutic drugs to the perforation site, optimizing effectiveness and reducing systemic adverse effects.

In addition, studies are looking at the potential therapeutic target of the microbiome as well as its involvement in the pathophysiology of gastrointestinal perforations. Perforations and related consequences have been linked to dysbiosis or an imbalance in the gut microbiota. Researchers hope to enhance patient outcomes for gastrointestinal perforation patients by restoring microbial equilibrium in the gut microbiome via the use of probiotics, prebiotics, or fecal microbiota transplantation.

Furthermore, current research in the area of gastrointestinal perforation continues to focus on improvements in surgical methods and tools. Researchers are always working to enhance the safety, effectiveness, and accessibility of treatment options for patients with perforated gastrointestinal disorders. This includes developing new endoscopic instruments for perforation closure and improving minimally invasive surgical techniques.

Clinicians and researchers aim to improve patient outcomes and quality of life by tackling these areas of ongoing research to deepen our understanding of gastrointestinal perforation and create novel approaches to its diagnosis, treatment, and prevention.

CONCLUSION

Finally, it should be noted that gastrointestinal perforations are serious medical conditions that may be fatal. This illness, which is defined by the development of a hole or rupture in the gastrointestinal system, has to be identified right once and treated very away. It has been clear from this discussion that several reasons, including internal medical disorders like ulcers, diverticulitis, or Crohn's disease, as well as external ones like trauma or surgical complications, may lead to the development of gastrointestinal perforation.

Gastrointestinal perforations may manifest clinically in a variety of ways, from minor stomach pain to severe sepsis and shock. Timely diagnosis is critical and often depends on a triage of laboratory tests, imaging tests (such as CT or X-rays), and clinical evaluation. Following diagnosis, treatment usually entails a multidisciplinary team of critical care doctors, surgeons, and gastroenterologists to stabilize the patient, manage sepsis, and repair the perforation using either non-surgical or surgical methods.

The patient's general health state, the degree of tissue damage, the promptness of management, and the underlying reason are some of the variables that affect the prognosis of gastrointestinal perforation. Although improvements in surgical methods and medical technology have led to better results over time, the death rate from gastrointestinal perforations is still high, particularly when there is insufficient or delayed treatment.

In conclusion, gastrointestinal perforation presents a serious clinical problem that has to be recognized quickly, diagnosed accurately, and treated promptly. Healthcare providers need to keep a close eye on patients who exhibit suggestive symptoms, especially if they have risk factors that predispose them to the condition. Healthcare professionals may improve patient outcomes and lessen the potentially disastrous effects of this critical medical illness by emphasizing early intervention and using a collaborative approach to patient care.

THE END